# Table of Contents

# The Relationship Between Body Image and Eating Disorders

# 1. Introduction to Body Image and Eating Disorders

This article first provides some definitions of terms that are used and then explores body image from various angles. We consider the prevalence of body image distortion and dissatisfaction, the likely precursors or predictors of poor body esteem, and the problems and consequences of body image disturbance. The subsequent part is critique and considers the limitations and strengths of the qualitative and quantitative approaches within body image research, highlighting the key areas in which they complement each other. We then trigger the development of a revision theory known as socio-cultural models. In this article, we critically review the literature pertaining to body image of women in midlife. The database PsycINFO was used to locate references pertaining to body image, midlife issues, and related concepts. The classification scheme for body image developed by Thompson and Stice was used to organize the review.

It is known that dissatisfaction with self-image is a risk factor for the onset and maintenance of eating disorders. Both women and men worry about their appearance; however, it is well documented that women are more dissatisfied with their physical appearance than men tend to be. Furthermore, pressure to conform to increasingly unrealistic standards of beauty may defy progress that has undoubtedly been made in media representation of natural body shapes. One excellent way to understand the factors that cause the onset and maintenance of eating disorders is to explore more deeply the role that body image disturbances play within the etiology. This article provides a critical overview of both quantitative and qualitative body image evidence in eating disorders. The importance of exploring the body image evidence is to inform the theoretical models that are most likely to predict and helpfully guide treatment strategies.

## 2. Understanding Body Image

People are heavily influenced by cultural ideals of beauty, images of which are unavoidable and presented in a variety of media. Women are particularly at risk as they have been socialized to equate attractiveness with thinness. Pitted against cultural standards, women question the value of achieving anything else if they are not physically desirable. Ideals of female beauty continue to emphasize thinness; and Hayes and Tantleff-Dunn report that the number of advertisements for makeovers and diet products (both of which focus on changing body shape and weight) proliferated in magazines since the early 1990s. Photographs of women in the 1920s in the New York Times showed homely women modeling undergarments, while contemporary images in a recent issue of Cosmopolitan feature taller, thinner, enormously improved women, glamour-girl outlines compared to loose girls. Body image is a psychological process that incorporates the cognitive or affective characteristics of body-related perceptions and includes a priori predispositions to surete training, diet and other health behaviors. The concept of body image is hierarchical with a relatively open definition at the top and more limited, clear, empirical, variables defining its aspects or factors. Central to body image is an individual's attractiveness.

Body image is a complex concept that refers to how individuals perceive and feel about their bodies. According to Thompson, body image incorporates "body-related perceptions," "body-related predispositions," and "body-related cognitive and affective experiences." In the field of representational practice, body image is used to refer mainly to "identity, social category, and self-perception." Gelder, Mayou, and Geddes argue that, in the context of psychopathology, body image simply refers to an "individual's concept of his own body." They stress that the concept of body image is imitative of that of body schema, a representation of our bodies in space. It refers to the various values individuals attribute to their appearance, attributions such as fat, small, ugly, sexy, and desirable. Inherent in body image is both a summary of and a projection into the future of one's life history. Given this conceptualization, there are several factors—through a variety of pathways—that influence the development of body image. These include: cultural ideals of beauty; social comparison processes; psychological variables; mediators; moderators; dieting; and genetics.

# 3. Types of Eating Disorders

All three eating disorders are very serious and can result in chronic medical conditions as a result of the sufferer's behavior. The two eating disorders, anorexia and bulimia, are the most common in teenage girls, and bulimia and binge eating disorder can be in teenage boys and young women. Noteworthy is the fact that most bulimics are very close to the normal weight, and the Hispanic community is more prone to develop this disorder. Most anorexics are in this range and a few overweight, and this disorder is more common in the Caucasian community. Early in a patient's pain, they may lose and gain similar 10 pounds in a few months and keep a standing weight. However, after a healthy body weight, a patient with bulimia nervosa may not achieve the level of weight loss as an anorexic patient, even though they are striving to starve all the time. As long as the patient with bulimia attempts purging, which includes vomiting, excessive excretion or the misuse of diuretics or laxatives, they can maintain a healthy body weight. On the other hand, like many anorexic patients, some who purge will lose their weight.

An eating disorder is a psychological illness that causes disturbances to its sufferer's everyday diet, which can manifest in the form of excessive eating or too little eating. Conversely, each eating disorder contains its own intertwined unique set of behaviors and thoughts. There are three most common types of eating disorders: anorexia nervosa, which is characterized by individual attempts to starve everything they consume into their bodies in achieving a goal; bulimia nervosa, where an individual might consume great quantities of food and then attempt to expel themselves of the calories, which can entail purging through vomiting using diuretics or weight loss, and excessive exercise as a means of body control; and binge-eating disorder, where an individual constantly eats beyond the point of feeling full, resulting in the individual becoming overweight or obese because they are eating such large amounts of food.

# 4. Causes and Risk Factors

The diathesis-stress model is the idea that the presence of a biological vulnerability predisposes a person to a pathological eating pattern and that exposure to certain environmental factors may result in the manifestation of an actual eating disorder.

Researchers have also shown that there are certain psychological factors that may increase an individual's risk of developing an eating disorder. A 2005 study showed that a negative body image has a direct link to the development of eating disorders. This may be true for children as well as adults, for women as well as for men. In addition, environmental factors like cultural pressures and the effects of the media may lead to the development of an eating disorder in some people. These influences can have a direct effect on individuals who are at risk for eating disorders, and the diathesis-stress model supports this.

The study of more than 31,000 female twins revealed that in the case of anorexia nervosa, genes accounted for about 56 percent of the cases of the disorder, while environmental factors accounted for about 44 percent. Additionally, some attempt to catalogue the possible risk factors, like genetics and personality, that contribute to the creation of eating disorders.

Although various underlying causes contribute to the development of eating disorders, the exact etiology is not known. Eating disorders are complex and influenced by both biological and environmental factors. Though the contribution of genetics to anorexia in particular is now accepted, a study suggests that environmental factors might play a heavier role in the development of eating disorders than previously thought.

# 5. Impact of Social Media and Society

It can also create a habit of frequently monitoring our own and others' bodies for any "flaws" and trigger eating disorder and exercise behaviors through comparison. Society can also have a direct impact which can be seen and felt after only a short period of time in a given country. In Fiji, a study of school girls had them self-reporting their desired body weight, before and after western television was introduced. They began to desire thinner bodies after a relatively short space of time. Even having knowledge of these influences might not be enough to stop someone from feeling dissatisfaction or engaging in these types of attitudes and behaviors. It is probable that a basic tenet of the way our brain operates works to compare ourselves to others for many different ends.

Another factor contributing to the rise of body dissatisfaction is the growing prevalence of social media. Engaging in social media has been linked with higher levels of body dissatisfaction and internalization of the thin-ideal among both men and women, suggesting that social media may have a profound impact on our body image. The media generally portrays a specific body type, which is idealized and rare, and can be both heavier or lighter than the healthier range for most people. As well as the portrayal of one type of body, there are a few other ways in which media may have an impact on our body image.

# 6. Recognizing Symptoms of Eating Disorders

Behavioral indicators of disordered eating: • Avoidance of social interactions (e.g. don't want to eat in front of people or in public food settings) • Defensiveness (especially about meal patterns or exercise habits) • Argue that they are "not that thin," even when BMI or weight loss shows to be underweight • Avoidance of judgments or evaluation concerning eating or body • Engage in secretive eating, hide food or eating patterns • Insist on eating alone because of "preference" or to work out, without evidence that they actually prefer this, or before/after a regular meal • A lack of change in body size appearance, when weight or size were "attacked" as perceived below satisfaction

Emotional indicators of disordered eating: • Anxiety • Depression or signs of sadness • Irritability • Emotional detachment • Lack of interest in previously pleasurable activities • Lack of attention or shifts in behavior indicating preoccupation (in general) with weight, size or body

Physical indicators of disordered eating: • Sudden or rapid weight loss or BMI drop • Sudden or rapid weight gain or BMI increase • Fainting, dizziness, nausea • Low energy level • Fatigue with no known cause • Hair loss with no known cause • Sensitivity to cold • Hypotension • Absent menses (for women) or hypomenorrhea • Gastrointestinal issues or pain • Excessive exercising • Dietary fasts (e.g. signs of extreme malnourishment)

Some possible signs and symptoms of a developing eating disorder are shown in this section. Note, if an individual is exhibiting these symptoms, it does not definitively mean the person has an eating disorder. There could be alternative explanations for sudden and significant weight changes, secretive eating or avoidance of particular foods, or excessive exercising. If you witness some or all of these symptoms, especially those in the physical category, this is an indication that the best thing you can do is communicate your concerns to a professional in the field of mental health. If you are especially close to the individual affected by suggestion of an eating disorder, it is necessary that this be brought to light with a person who can help.

# 7. When to Seek Professional Help

Additionally, if you eat a lot of food in a very short period of time and feel a loss of control and intense distress before or after you binge, you may be struggling with binge eating, which signals that it is important to seek help. An eating disorder, if left untreated, can have serious, life-threatening consequences, including a 12-fold increase in premature death, severe health consequences (e.g. bone density loss, digestive problems, heart conditions), and higher rates of depression and anxiety. Although reliable statistics are hard to come by, current estimates for recovery from eating disorders are in the range of 30-50% for various diagnoses. It is crucial to seek help immediately in these cases since professional treatment can greatly increase the likelihood of recovery. Evidence shows it is much easier to treat what could be considered sub-clinical symptoms or general concerns about weight and body shape than it is to address a full-blown eating disorder.

It is important to seek professional help if an eating disorder is negatively affecting various aspects of your life, such as physical health or mental and emotional well-being. A trained professional can help address issues, identify underlying causes, and suggest appropriate treatments. General signs that you can look for (and that are often used to diagnose eating disorders) include severely restricted food intake, ongoing worrying about food and weight, and constant dieting, regardless of body size. These symptoms can be associated with body weight changes and can manifest in physical symptoms including short-term signs of starvation (e.g. slow heart rate, reduced blood pressure), fatigue, or irregular menstruation.

# 8. Treatment Options for Eating Disorders

Treatment for eating disorders typically involves a variety of professionals, each with a different area of expertise relevant to eating disorders. Several areas may need attention, including medical, psychological, and nutritional. The treatment plan depends on the unique situation of the individual. There might be one primary therapist who coordinates the consultations and treatments with other professionals, or an individual might be involved with different professionals separately. Often, family members are also involved in treatment to achieve the best outcomes, especially for children and adolescents. Personal attitude towards treatment is the most important factor in determining whether someone might recover from an eating disorder. Success in both reducing disordered eating symptoms and in maintaining them to achieve a return to a healthier lifestyle is not simply about identifying 'the best' treatment option, but rather is about finding the best fit between an individual and particular intervention strategies to manage disorder symptoms. A combination of approaches seems to have the best results.

The treatments for eating disorders vary according to the diagnosis and the severity of the disorder. They may include inpatient, outpatient, or day programs to provide medical monitoring, nutritional rehabilitation, and support for psychological and behavioral changes. A range of services might become involved as needed, including physicians, mental health professionals, dietitians, and social workers. The ultimate goal in the treatment of eating disorders is to treat all aspects of the disorder. Below is a description of modalities and interventions sometimes employed in treating eating disorders.

# 9. Prevention Strategies and Self-Care

While fixing individuals or the thin ideal are not realistic nor particularly helpful long-term solutions, preventing the development of an eating disorder usually involves decades of concerted public health effort and focus. To be effective, prevention strategies are integrated, evidence-based approaches that are applied at a number of different levels: to the individual, to parents and families, to schools and teachers, and to the broader community as a whole. Strategy areas include promoting a positive body image, offering education and guidance on improving and maintaining good mental health, as well as counseling and psychological services when appropriate. Some common prevention advice is on healthier eating and physical activity.

2. Prevention Strategies

Regular exercise can form part of a largely positive impact on body image. People who exercise frequently are more likely to think of themselves as attractive and are less likely to experience extreme dissatisfaction with their appearance. However, people who exercise to change the way they look, or become preoccupied with the shape of their body, can jeopardize the benefits they receive from exercise for their body and mind.

1. Self-Care

Everybody can play a role in reducing the risk of developing an eating disorder, both for themselves and for their friends, family, and colleagues. In order to break free from the narrow perceptions the common portrayal of eating disorders allows for, this understanding involves a recognition of widespread weight and shape concerns - and a general absence of satisfaction with personal appearances - as an integral element of the modern condition for many.

# 10. Supporting a Loved One with an Eating Disorder

You can provide a safe and supportive environment for the person involved. Once the person feels understood and supported, they are more likely to reach out for help. You do not need to try a 'cure' for the person. You are not responsible for their recovery. It is their responsibility. At times, you might feel unsure of what to do and who to talk to about the best ways of helping the person who has an eating disorder. The person may have talked to you now and I suggest you talk to someone you trust who can help and support you. There are many support groups for family and friends, many of which provide over-the-phone support. It is important that you have people to talk to about how you are going as well.

Support is extremely important to recovery. Many people feel uncomfortable when trying to help a friend or family member who has an eating disorder. They may not know how to talk about it or may be worried about upsetting the person with the eating disorder. It can feel like a huge relief for the person with an eating disorder to finally talk about it. The person is letting you know, as a friend, that they trust you. This could be a voice coming from their recovery. The person with an eating disorder does not expect friends and family to be able to fix them.

# 11. Conclusion and Future Directions

It is apparent that males tend not to show the degree of body dissatisfaction shown by females. However, recent extreme male dieters with eating disordered psychopathology (alongside females) continued to show a cognitively biased body image. However, little body dissatisfaction was evidenced in a true male comparison group. The universal problem of failing to be able to control one's weight has therefore been a target of study for the general population, dieters, and across medical and psychological populations. The intervention study has preliminarily shown that it is possible to change people's cognitive biases in regard to their body size estimation in the population and men. The direction for future research would include long-term follow-up on the interview study to see who has developed eating disordered psychopathology and to replicate the intervention study in a true eating disordered group. It would also be informative to compare the body image of people who have lost weight and gained it back again, to those who have lost weight and kept it off. It would also be informative to do the studies investigating body satisfaction, body change attempts, and body shape estimation in an eating disordered male sample. In short, this research has greatly contributed to understanding the complex relationships associated with body image and eating disordered populations on many levels and in each mooted future direction. The evidence supports that future research in this field of eating disorders is warranted and required.

This essay has comprehensively presented an exploration of the relationships between body image and eating disorders. More specifically, it has reviewed multiple aspects addressing body image disturbances in relation to eating disordered populations. These have included body dissatisfaction across various diagnostic categories, weight loss attempts and success, body image disturbances from all areas of body image, alternate body image measures, and investigating more extreme dieters with eating disordered psychopathology (although many more mildly eating disordered individuals were included in the studies). These themes were examined in relation to various populations and with different research designs, including investigating the information available through population studies and self-reports of body image. More recently, this research has been grounded in cognitive-behavioral theory using more experimental designs to investigate body image self-schema. Preliminary and replicated results showed a clear relationship between cognitive errors in body shape misperception on a body size estimation task.

Concluding comments

# The Relationship Between Body Image and Disordered Eating Habits

# 1. Introduction to Body Image and Disordered Eating

This essay will explore the relationship between body dissatisfaction and disordered eating. Specific areas of exploration will include: historical trends in body perception and chronic dieting; the influence of the weight loss industry and objectification theory on a woman's attempts to reach societal expectations; and the role of biological factors related to a woman's struggle with disordered eating and body image.

The idea of a woman with a body fat percentage as low as seven percent starving and endangering her life by spending three hours at the gym because she believes she is morbidly obese may seem absurd. However, this is happening to young women at increasingly younger ages. Research suggests that as many as 65% of American women report disordered eating behaviors and symptoms. It is clear that negative body image and disordered eating need to be examined. This phenomenon centers not only on an individual woman, but also an entire society, permeating fairy tales, films, magazines, family members, peers, and the medical community.

## 2. The Impact of Media and Societal Standards on Body Image

The media is an influential part of everyday life, which contributes to negative body image and promotes unhealthy relationships with food. The "body image" that individuals hold of themselves can be influenced by their physical and social environment. One of the areas within the social context that has been said to contribute to an individual's body dissatisfaction is the media. With today's society being dominated by mass media as a popular form of entertainment, information, and communication, the media is a powerful tool used to influence cultural, societal, and personal values. In fact, bodies that are portrayed as being "capable, undisciplined, 'less' fat, or non-fat in the media are portrayed in ways that are not typically very positive.

Despite the common belief that body image is developed intrinsically and from inner values, studies have shown an effect from both mass media and societal standards in promoting body dissatisfaction and disordered eating patterns across cultures. This section of the paper aims to understand how exposure and access to media representations of the body may influence individuals' perceptions of the body. Using thin ideals displayed in different media forms, including advertising and popular culture, this part of the paper may also examine how repeatedly viewing these unrealistic portrayals contributes to negative body image and a strained relationship with food.

# 3. Psychological Factors Influencing Body Image Perception

Attending to the prior comments, this work is directed towards introducing those factors contributing to the development of disordered eating habits. This may provide better knowledge of some elements contributing to their psychopathological features. The third section of this paper focuses on the psychological factors determining body image perception. Relevant literature shows that self-esteem is inversely related to body dissatisfaction. Some studies have shown that pre-adolescents already predisposed to dissatisfaction with their figure have worse health habits than people without low body acceptance. These people are consequently likely to suffer from metabolic syndromes. Moreover, in the 1950s terms such as self-image, body-image, or body-schema appeared to explain the variability in human perception of their appearance. These terms reflect the anatomical place situation in the 3D-schema, perceived by the subject. If the stereotype of the body is inadequate, then dysmorphophobia can occur. Dysmorphophobia is characterized by obsessions or compulsions related to one or more imperfections in appearance. This, in turn, can lead to mood problems, such as anxiety and depression. The term "self-schema" identifies an individual assessment of oneself, such as gender, nationality, religion, etc. Riegele in 1940 defined it as an indicator of the emotional attitude of people towards themselves. Men show a perennial and multifaceted relationship with their physical image (male body image) as well. Men and women want to be slender: the Cult of the thin ideal: examples of the thin-culture model are found in advertising, magazines, television, and movies. The psychological mechanisms responsible for altered body image perception are unclear. There is probably a combination of cognitive processes, based on attention and evaluation, and emotional factors, which could contribute to the development of selective information processing. Moreover, some individual psychological traits are able to determine the development of body image perception. These personality traits can lead to eating disorders because they increase concerns about body weight, feelings of inadequateness, and fear of getting fat. No epidemiological research of delusional dysmorphophobia has been conducted in Italy. Women are generally more concerned with their appearance than men. The studies showed that 25% of women have significant concerns about their appearance. Concern about body image is closely related to eating habits and metabolism.

Body image perception reflects how a person views his or her body. It is influenced by both physiological and psychological factors. Female and/or male disordered body image perception is a superficial and pathological point of view about their figure, body weight, and a desire to change any of them. The incidence of these abnormal feelings about the physical aspect in adolescence can lead to serious mental disorders, such as eating disorders, including anorexia, bulimia, and Binge Eating Disorders

(BED). The cause of altered body image perception might be identified in the interaction among various factors, such as cultural habitus, stress, a deficiency in coping strategies, personality features, and biological factors. Furthermore, food, eating, and body weight gain are surrounded by the importance of psychological meanings, which might profoundly influence the mental system.

# 4. Types of Disordered Eating Habits and Eating Disorders

Diagnostic criteria for specific types of eating disorders overlap, but there are also key symptoms and behavioral expectations that individualize the diagnoses. AN is subtyped as either restricting type, in which weight gain is prevented through dieting, fasting, and excessive exercise, or as binge eating/purge type, which is differentiated from bulimia nervosa (BN) by the degree of emaciation. AN is diagnosed when a person has a body mass index (BMI) of ≤17.5 kg/m, denies the seriousness of low body weight, has amenorrhea, and has an intense fear of weight gain or becoming fat OR when an individual has low body weight due to recurrent binge eating and purging behavior.

The concept of disordered eating encompasses various eating behaviors that can be characterized as unrealistic or excessive, maladaptive, or even bizarre. Disordered eating habits can be viewed on a continuum and can range from normal but intense dieting behavior to severe food-abuse syndromes. This spectrum includes various forms and degrees of food restriction, such as chronic dieting, subclinical and clinical anorexia nervosa (AN), partial syndrome anorexia nervosa (PSAN), and subthreshold anorexia nervosa, which are not officially part of the Diagnostic and Statistical Manual of Mental Disorders, Fourth Edition, Text Revision (DSM-IV-TR) criteria. Disordered eating involves restriction and binge eating behaviors that result from an over-evaluation of shape and weight. Together, voluntary dieting and restrained eating have been popularly referred to as "disordered eating," including individuals who are preoccupied with dieting and obsessed with food. Disordered eating behavior is not diagnosed and treated as an eating disorder. This group with subclinical eating disorder cases is often called "disordered eating" and includes many women.

# 5. Anorexia Nervosa: Symptoms, Causes, and Treatment

The sufferer can also experience depression, anxiety, and displacement disorder. There is a lack of emotion and concentration can be low. Anxiety, mood swings, and aggressiveness are also frequent. Tremors are often present. A high resting heart rate is a sign that a patient suffering from anorexia is underweight and is a sign of anorexia nervosa. The pulse may be faint and the pain may be severe. It is the conscious fear of gaining weight and becoming fat, despite being seriously underweight. In most cases, anorexia is due to multiple factors, and in some cases, psychological therapy, nutritional therapy, and medication are required. Treatment can help, but it is not a cure. If used after being diagnosed with anorexia, it can give you more physical and mental problems, so you won't recover and can lead to preventable complications or it will just return over and over again.

Anorexia nervosa is an eating disorder which can be associated with a distorted body image, obsession with food and calorie intake. Individuals suffering from anorexia may experience one or more psychological or behavioral symptoms: starving oneself, repeated weighing of oneself, yellowing of the skin, self-induced vomiting, stick-thin appearance, worn tooth enamel, and thin appearance or weakness.

# 6. Bulimia Nervosa: Symptoms, Causes, and Treatment

Bulimia may be well hidden by the person with the illness, and it is often only those closest to that individual who will be aware that there is anything wrong. Eating disorders are known to have begun somewhere between the ages of 15 and 25, but it can start at any time in life and affects 1-2% of adolescents and young women. Recovery from the eating disorder can take years, and even then many never fully recover. The use of formal treatment, for example, including antipsychotic medication and/or psychotherapy, can increase recovery rates. Generally, healthy and normal weight people with bulimia nervosa often have an overvalued idea of the importance of weight/shape and are intensely unhappy with their size and body shape. Management for bulimia nervosa has been researched in numerous randomized control treatment studies, and two forms of psychotherapy treatment are now known to work: manual-based cognitive-behavioral treatment and interpersonal psychotherapy.

Bulimia nervosa is a common eating disorder that was first described in the 1980s. It is characterized by a number of symptoms, perhaps the most recognizable of which is binge eating or eating an excessive amount of food in a short time. This is followed by one or more ways of getting rid of the food just eaten, such as forced vomiting, excessive use of laxatives or diuretics, or excessive exercise. There is a sense of loss of control over the binge eating and safety amnesia in important aspects of life and judgment. Bulimia nervosa can possess many features of other conditions, such as depression, schizophrenia, or personality disorders. It may also be associated with talkative behavior or impulsivity in some people. People with bulimia nervosa are usually normal weight or slightly overweight.

# 7. Binge Eating Disorder: Characteristics and Interventions

Characteristic of binge eating episodes, individuals commonly report feeling shame, disgust, and guilt. Often described as an escape or outlet, individuals tend to use the episodes as a means to "lose themselves" or to gain relief from stressors. The lack of successful resolution of the stressor, however, is problematic and leads to repeated and persistent episodes of abnormal food intake behaviors. Individuals with BED also report feelings of physical discomfort, fullness, and expect compensation from restricting food, purging, or exercising to relieve the pressure or reduce the possibility of weight gain. Additionally, binge eating episodes trigger feelings of low self-esteem, sadness, and dissatisfaction with body shape.

Labeled as the "new" eating disorder in the Diagnostic and Statistical Manual of Mental Disorders' fourth edition (DSM-IV), binge eating disorder (BED) was noted as an area deserving of additional research. Since the publication of that edition, substantial progress has been made in the understanding of this excessive consumption condition. The successor to this edition, DSM-5, now includes separate diagnostic criteria for BED, which substantiates its existence as a clinical syndrome. Primarily identified by episodes of consuming an unusually large amount of food in a discrete period of time and experiencing a loss of control, individuals with BED often engage in episodes of extreme caloric consumption that are perceived as an "emotional outlet and escape." After engaging in a binge, individuals may feel distressed, remorseful, guilty, disgusted, ashamed, or generally regretful. This cycle of binge eating and consequential negative emotions can hold an iron grip on individuals, consuming their thoughts and focus, leading to time being taken up by thought processes concerning food, body, exercise, and plans for strategies to control eating that need not intersect a binge, such as exercise regimens, dieting, and the avoidance of weight gain strategies. Most bitter of all, these approaches ultimately fail to alleviate feelings of low self-esteem, sadness, and dissatisfaction with life, just as the previous binge-eating episodes hadn't.

Kirsty M. Daniels, Caroline Davis, Richard A. Kuehne, and J. Kevin Thompson.

# 8. Body Dysmorphic Disorder and its Relation to Eating Disorders

There is frequently a longitudinal link between body image disturbance and disordered eating, in which body dysmorphia maintains the eating disorder and vice versa. This relationship is complex, and there is still a great deal of guesswork into the causative factors, possible routes of development, and necessary intervention at initial stages. The assessment and treatment of body image disturbance have been of interest due to the impingement on individuals' quality of life across various areas of function, and the impact on the development and maintenance of eating disorders. Yet, as a symptom that is not necessary for an eating disorder to be diagnosable, several affected individuals fall through the gap without appropriate care and intervention. Interventions need to be tailored to the individual's specific needs and driven by a model which effectively illustrates the individual pathway and the development of causative factors.

Finally, it is worth discussing the concept of body dysmorphic disorder (BDD) and its relation to eating disorders, while noting that this does not reflect those with identified BDD. BDD is distinguished by an obsessive preoccupation with perceived flaws in physical appearance. This, too, may be applicable to a certain extent in the context of eating disorders, as individuals may suffer from apparent inaccuracies in conceptualizing body size and shape. There is evidence to suggest that excessive attention to shape could be a causative feature of eating disorders. Anderson and Thompson's Strengths and Weaknesses of the DSM-5 level of implementation criteria for feeding or eating disorders provide a useful insight into the debates surrounding the diagnostic criteria for eating disorder subtypes.

# 9. Intersectionality and Body Image: The Role of Race, Gender, and Sexual Orientation

Body image encompasses our conceptualization of our physical self – it includes personal views about our body size, form, height, weight, and our understanding about our physical self in relation to others. Our culture places large focuses on body image, and many individuals spend a lot of time trying to change their weights, shapes, or forms. Research has shown that overall, body dissatisfaction is associated with disordered eating attitudes and/or acts. Indeed, research with women has shown that disordered eating rate scores declined when the level of body dissatisfaction decreased, and men who were more dissatisfied with their bodies also reported greater drive for muscularity. Hence, for many people, the concentrated effort to look a particular way does correlate with disordered eating attitudes, beliefs, and subsequently, behavior. In sum, body dissatisfaction seems to be important when understanding disordered eating, and this study adds to the literature by showing that in fact, theory regarding Social Comparison is relevant to men of diverse orientations.

Body image is a complex issue, and how we perceive our bodies can be shaped by societal rules and regulations. In turn, our personal perceptions of ourselves can impact the way we engage with the world. Intersectionality is the understanding that individuals face multiple forces of oppression including race, gender, sexual orientation, and ability. Taking an intersectional approach to body image, we explore the idea that for women and men of different racial backgrounds, the societal pressures to fit into a particular body image 'ideal' differ. This section will help you understand the different experiences individuals may have about their body image and potential disordered eating habits due to the myriad of factors that collide in any given individual's life.

# 10. Prevention and Intervention Strategies for Disordered Eating

There are a number of interventions at various levels that have been found to lead to improvements in body image and eating disorder behaviors such as disordered eating and unhealthy weight control strategies. Most approaches to bulimia or binge eating involve addressing the underlying problem to prevent the individual from using food as a dysfunctional coping strategy. These are a form of cognitive-behavioral therapy (CBT). However, other psychological therapies cannot only help people to overcome disordered eating but can also raise awareness and challenge some of the wider pressure (e.g., media) and cultural body image norms. Several prevention and early intervention programs have been found to reduce risk factors for and prevent disordered eating in young people. Programs that have been found to be effective tend to be based on promoting wider messages of healthy eating and a healthy body image, and suggest ways to adopt regular eating patterns and pay attention to the hunger and fullness signals from the body.

Prevention and early intervention efforts for individuals at risk of developing disordered eating-related behaviors, including body image issues, should generally target proximal, individualized causes of disordered eating, such as appearance pressures and the disruption of normal hunger and fullness cues, as well as those related to eating disorder behaviors as coping strategies. One study showed that individual-based prevention to groups of adolescents at risk for eating and weight concerns moderated some of the proximal appearance, eating behavior, and weight-related risk factors from pre- to post-intervention. Systemic (e.g., policy) and environmental (e.g., school or university ground) prevention constitute more of a primary prevention approach that potentially influences whole societies.

# 11. The Importance of Early Detection and Treatment

The impact of detection and treatment at an early stage on disordered eating habits and onset of full-blown eating disorders is extensively described. The psychological distress incurred at early stages is higher when pathways are not changed due to overt preoccupation with weight and shape, dieting, food restriction, strong dispositional conditions for developing an eating disorder, a desire for thinness, and low self-esteem that predict the most severe (or even incurable) eating disorders. It is only by putting the full scope of diagnoses aside, and by being sensitive to earlier signs and distress, that we can hope for a broader amelioration of the problem— both for individuals and society.

Early in the development of an eating disorder, the function behind the disordered eating act is difficult to recognize because the disturbing habits are often hidden behind what appears to be a regular or accepted behavior. As the eating disorder and disordered thinking process around food, weight, or body image becomes more complex, the attainment of a healthy body image and eating habits increasingly diminishes; yet the habit of disordered eating may have already become ingrained. The consequences of leaving individuals to struggle with disordered eating judged only by the severity of a likely diagnosable eating disorder is disturbing. While trauma experienced during bouts of illness may activate the intervention of mental health services, many others may not develop an illness severe enough to warrant immediate treatment. Consequently, these individuals are not provided with resources to help put an end to their misery.

# 12. Body Positivity Movements and Their Impact

While body positivity movements set out with the intention of promoting positive regard for bodies and emphasizing the limitations of physical appearance in determining one's worth, the potential exists for these messages to be undermining. In particular, because of the emphasis on appreciation and love of one's body, failure to internalize these views is subject to blame on a personal level, mistaking attitudinal change for affective change. Attitudes often follow affect, and therefore proffering "positive" attitudes toward all bodies will do little to change individuals' self-perception. Having a better understanding of the impact of body positivity movements as a discourse is important for advancing our knowledge on how to best interact with individuals and yet focus on these structural factors rather than the purely individual level.

In recent years, there has been increasing societal attention and acknowledgment of the importance of promoting a positive body image among individuals in order to mitigate the development of disordered eating habits. A common form of cultural focus in this area has been with the rise of body positivity movements. Discussions of body satisfaction often seem to stem from statistics that focus on the thin ideal in the United States and the narrow window of socially acceptable body types. From a public health standpoint, however, suggesting better psychological health can come from promoting a few more cups of kale and a little more time on the treadmill is not only physiologically inaccurate but also harmful.

# 13. Research and Studies on Body Image and Eating Disorders

The available literature suggests that there is a correlation between body dissatisfaction and disordered eating. The study aimed to first examine to what extent body dissatisfaction is able to predict both total eating disordered behaviors and the specific behaviors of eating disordered mentality, dieting intentions and behaviors, pressure to be thin, and societal pressure to be thin. Secondly, it was hypothesized that individuals who have been diagnosed with having an eating disorder will indicate a significantly higher level of body dissatisfaction than individuals without an eating disorder. This study supports previous research that attitude and concerns of body and self are associated with disordered eating. One's general displeasure with their body is a better predictor of eating behaviors than each of the component questions. These findings are important because the risk for dieting and eating problems appears earlier in the college years. Further, intervention tactics or strategies that are supportive of these findings should be enacted in the college health centers, where our at-risk subjects were located.

These four sources are specifically based on researching the relationship between body image and disordered eating. In each source, the body image and its relevance to disordered eating are examined. Each source also reports that body image is correlated positively with disordered eating. It is of current knowledge that there exists a relationship between body dissatisfaction and disordered eating habits. Studies have gone to investigate the occurrence of disordered eating amongst the individuals with clinical and non-clinical disorder. This study aims to provide the one final result by studying the concept in reference to the college student population and the Texas population to provide a clearer understanding of body image and its relation to disordered eating. And since there is evidence to support a relationship, it would be beneficial to concentrate on intervention techniques supportive in these specific areas of disorder that can help educate individuals on developing a healthier overall self-concept and body image perceptions.

# 14. Conclusion and Future Directions

Our understanding of the relationship between body image and disordered eating is becoming more sophisticated. Despite the evidence to support the complex relationship between body image and disordered eating, there is still much to learn and untangle. Areas for future research include extending the limited body image protective factor research to focus on protective factors for negative male body image eating and body image protective factors for samples with clinical eating disorder populations. Other areas for future research involve trialing interventions that target negative body image and low self-esteem to ascertain if this is a successful secondary prevention strategy that can reduce disordered eating, and examining primary prevention utilities. Further examining the relationship between body image and physical activity and sports is also required. Addressing negative body image and resultant eating disturbances and prevention strategies are also important advocacy and practice priorities.

Research examining the development of negative body image contributing to disordered eating focuses attention towards prevention and intervention strategies to assist those struggling with poor body image and disordered eating thoughts and behaviors. This includes considerations for promoting positive and healthy body image, empowering self-acceptance, addressing issues of body dissatisfaction and body objectification, and reducing thin-ideal internalization and celebrating body diversity.

A positive body image, characterized by contentment, self-acceptance, and appreciation for one's healthy body, is a vital protective factor against disordered eating. Negative body image, characterized by a focus on body dissatisfaction and distortion, contributes to the pathogenesis and persistence of disordered eating behaviors. Body image and eating disturbances have complex and multifactorial relationships, primarily explained through sociocultural, psychological, familial, and biological theories.